COMPLETE GUIDE TO GASTROESOPHAGEAL REFLUX DISEASE

Comprehensive Insights To Understanding, Managing, Preventing, Treatments, And Diet Tips For Long-Term Relief

DEHART HAIRSTON

© [DEHART HAIRSTON], [2024]

All rights reserved. No part of this publication may be reproduced, distributed, or transmitted in any form or by any means, including photocopying, recording, or other electronic or mechanical methods, without the prior written permission of the publisher, except in the case of brief quotations embodied in critical reviews and certain other noncommercial uses permitted by copyright law.

DISCLAIMER

This book's content is only intended for general informative purposes. At the time of writing, the author has taken every precaution to guarantee that the material is correct and current. Nevertheless, the author disclaims all explicit and implicit representations and guarantees about the availability, appropriateness, correctness, completeness, and usefulness of the material on these pages.

Since the author is not a licensed medical practitioner, the material in this book shouldn't be interpreted as medical advice. Before making any modifications to their diet, exercise regimen, or medical treatment, readers are urged to speak with a licensed healthcare provider.

Moreover, the author has no connection to any of the businesses, organizations, or people that are discussed in this book. Any mentions of goods, services, businesses, or people are purely informative and do not indicate endorsement or suggestion.

This book's content is entirely dependent on the author's expertise, study, and comprehension of the topic. Despite having taken reasonable care to offer correct information, the author disclaims all liability for any mistakes or omissions in the material as well as for any losses, harm, or damages resulting from using the information.

It is recommended that readers use their own judgment and discretion when applying the knowledge in this book to their own situations. The use or implementation of any material in this book may result in unfavorable repercussions, directly or indirectly, for which the author assumes no liability.

By reading this book, you agree to release and hold the author harmless from any claims, losses, liabilities, costs, or expenditures resulting from or related to the use of the information you get from it.

Table of Contents

CHAPTER 1 15
Understanding Gastroesophageal Reflux Disease (GERD) 15
What Is GERD? 15
Causes And Risk Factors 16
- • Hiatal Hernia: 16
- • Obesity: 16
- • Specific Foods and Drinks: 16
- • Smoking: 17
- • Pregnancy: 17
- • Certain medicines: 17

Symptoms And Diagnosis 18
- • Heartburn: 18
- • Regurgitation: 18
- • Dysphagia: 18
- • Chronic Cough: 18
- • Hoarseness or Sore Throat: 18

CHAPTER 2 21
Anatomy Of Gerd 21
How The Digestive System Works 21

- The Role Of The Esophagus And Lower Esophageal Sphincter (Les) 22
- Mechanisms Of Reflux 24

CHAPTER 3 27
- Lifestyle Modifications For Managing Gerd 27
- Dietary Changes: Foods To Avoid And Foods To Include 27
  - Foods to Steer Clear of: 27
  - Foods to Add: 29
- Importance Of Weight Management 30
  - How Losing Weight Benefits: 31
- Tips For Eating And Drinking 32
  - Tips for Eating: 32
  - Tips for Drinking: 33

CHAPTER 4 35
- Medications For Gerd 35
- Over-The-Counter Antacids 35
- H2 Receptor Blockers 36
- Proton Pump Inhibitors (Ppis) 38

CHAPTER 5 43
- Surgical Options For Gerd 43
- Fundoplication Surgery 43

- Endoscopic Treatments 45
- Patient Selection And Risks 47

CHAPTER 6 49
- Complications Of Untreated Gerd 49
- Esophagitis And Barrett's Esophagus 49
- Strictures And Ulcers 50
- Respiratory Complications 52

CHAPTER 7 54
- Gerd In Special Populations 54
- Gerd In Pregnancy 54
- Gerd In Children 56
- Gerd In The Elderly 58

CHAPTER 8 61
- Managing Gerd Symptoms 61
- Tips For Nighttime Heartburn Relief 61
  1. Raise Your Upper Extremities: 61
  2. Prevent Eating Late at Night: 61
  3. Adjust Your Position While Sleeping: 62
  4. Keep an Eye on Your Prescriptions: 62
  5. Determine Food Triggers: 62
  6. Utilize relaxation techniques: 63

Coping With Regurgitation And Chest Pain 63
- 1. Sustain a Healthy Weight: 64
- 2. Put on loose-fitting attire: 64
- 3. Steer clear of trigger foods: 64
- 4. Consume More Often and Smaller Meals: 65
- 5. Maintain Proper Posture: 65
- 6. Maintain Hydration: 65

Alleviating Throat Symptoms 66
- 1. Steer clear of irritants: 66
- 2. Maintain Hydration: 66
- 3. Employ a Humidifier: 67
- 4. Maintain Proper Oral Hygiene: 67
- 5. Avert Clearing Your Throat: 67
- 6. Think About Over-the-Counter Treatments: .. 68

CHAPTER 9 69
Integrative Approaches To Gerd Management 69
Supplements and Herbal Remedies 69
Stress Reduction Techniques 71
Alternative Therapies 73

CHAPTER 10: 75

Preventing Gerd Flare-Ups And Long-Term Management 75

Developing A Personalized Management Plan 75

Follow-Up Care And Monitoring 78

Living Well With Gerd: Tips For Long-Term Health 80

CONCLUSION 84

THE END 87

ABOUT THE BOOK

"Gastroesophageal Reflux Disease" is a valuable resource for anybody suffering from GERD or looking for in-depth knowledge on how to treat it. It's not simply another book about medical ailments. This book delves into the complexities of GERD and provides a plethora of information essential for comprehending the disease's anatomy, available treatments, and long-term management techniques.

The groundwork is laid in Chapter 1, which explains the basics of GERD and explains its origins, symptoms, and methods of diagnosis. This is an essential overview that makes sure readers understand the basics of the condition before going further.

Next, Chapter 2 delves into the anatomy at play, explaining the functions of the digestive system and the significance of important parts like the esophagus and lower esophageal sphincter. Gaining an understanding of these processes is essential to understanding reflux dynamics and its consequences.

In-depth strategies for treating GERD are covered in Chapters 3 and 4, including dietary changes, lifestyle changes, and the use of drugs such as proton pump inhibitors and antacids. With the help of this useful advice, people are better equipped to take charge of their health and improve their quality of life.

In addition to helping readers through the decision-making process and outlining possible risks and advantages, Chapter 5 provides essential insights into the range of alternatives accessible to people thinking about surgical procedures.

Beyond the fundamentals, the book discusses the consequences of untreated GERD, and how it affects certain demographics such as the elderly, children, and pregnant women, and provides advice on how to manage symptoms and avoid flare-ups.

In Chapter 9, integrative approaches to managing GERD are presented. It is acknowledged that herbal medicines, stress-reduction methods, and alternative therapies may be beneficial in addition to traditional treatments.

Ultimately, Chapter 10 makes sure readers have the information and resources they need to successfully navigate their path to optimum health by highlighting the significance of long-term strategies and customized management plans for living well with GERD.

"Gastroesophageal Reflux Disease" is an essential tool for everyone suffering from GERD since, at its core, it is not simply a book but also a road map for comprehending, treating, and eventually curing the illness.

CHAPTER 1

Understanding Gastroesophageal Reflux Disease (GERD)

What Is GERD?

The chronic digestive condition known as gastroesophageal reflux disease (GERD) is characterized by the reflux of stomach acid into the esophagus, the tube that runs from your mouth to your stomach. The lower esophageal sphincter (LES), a ring of muscle, normally functions as a valve to stop stomach acid from rising and entering the esophagus. But in people with GERD, this valve weakens or relaxes abnormally, letting stomach acid escape and causing esophageal irritation and inflammation.

Causes And Risk Factors

Although the precise etiology of GERD is not always known, several variables may play a role in its development. One main contributing aspect is the LES's weakening, which may happen for several reasons, including:

- Hiatal Hernia: A disorder in which part of the stomach pushes on the LES by protruding through the diaphragm and into the chest cavity.

- Obesity: Being overweight may raise abdominal pressure, which can cause the contents of the stomach to rise into the esophagus.

- Specific Foods and Drinks: Alcohol, caffeine, and carbonated drinks, along with spicy, fatty, or acidic foods, may relax the LES or irritate the esophagus, worsening symptoms.

- **Smoking:** Smoking weakens the LES and reduces salivation, which typically balances stomach acid.

- **Pregnancy:** During pregnancy, there are hormonal changes that might relax the LES and raise intrauterine pressure, which can result in GERD symptoms.

- **Certain medicines:** By relaxing the LES or irritating the esophagus, certain medicines, including calcium channel blockers, nonsteroidal anti-inflammatory drugs (NSAIDs), and several asthma treatments, may aggravate GERD.

Aside from these variables, other risk factors for GERD include age, genetics, and specific medical diseases including gastroparesis or scleroderma.

Symptoms And Diagnosis

A wide range of symptoms, varying in intensity from person to person, might be indicative of GERD. Typical signs and symptoms include:

- Heartburn: A burning feeling in the chest that usually happens at night or after eating.

- Regurgitation: The feeling of food or acid resurfacing in the mouth or throat.

- Dysphagia: The inability to swallow or the feeling that food is lodged in the throat.

- Chronic Cough: A chronic cough caused by stomach acid irritating the throat, which is usually worse at night or after eating.

- Hoarseness or Sore Throat: Acid reflux-related irritation of the vocal cords or throat tissue.

- Asthma: In some people, GERD may exacerbate asthma symptoms or precipitate asthma episodes.

A combination of the patient's medical history, physical examination, and diagnostic testing is usually used to diagnose GERD. Your symptoms, food habits, lifestyle choices, and any drugs you are taking may all be questioned by your doctor. To check for any indications of problems or underlying diseases, they could also do a physical examination.

GERD diagnostic testing may include the following in addition to a complete history and physical examination:

- Upper endoscopy: A technique in which the stomach and esophagus are visually inspected and, if required, tissue samples are taken using a thin, flexible tube equipped with a camera.

- Esophageal pH Monitoring: This test uses a tiny probe that is put via the nose into the esophagus to monitor the amount of acid present in the esophagus over the course of 24 hours.

• Esophageal Manometry: This test may be used to assess how well the LES and esophageal muscles are functioning by measuring the pressure and synchronization of muscular contractions in the esophagus.

These diagnostic procedures assist in determining if GERD is present, gauging its severity, and ruling out other illnesses that may cause comparable symptoms. Treatment for GERD may be customized to control symptoms and avoid problems after a diagnosis.

CHAPTER 2

Anatomy Of Gerd

How The Digestive System Works

Comprehending the digestive tract is essential to appreciating the intricacies of gastroenteritis. Imagine it as a well-oiled machine, where every component is essential to the process of nutrient absorption and food breakdown. Everything starts in the mouth, where salivary enzymes initiate the chemical digestive process, and chewing initiates the mechanical breakdown of food.

Food passes down the esophagus, a muscular tube that connects the neck and stomach, once it has been swallowed. By serving as a bridge, the esophagus directs food to its proper location. The esophagus is vulnerable to injury when exposed to stomach acid for prolonged periods, as in the case of GERD, since it is not made to tolerate the acidic environment found in the stomach.

The Lower Esophageal Sphincter (LES), a ring of muscle near the end of the esophagus that serves as a barrier between the esophagus and the stomach, is located there. The LES opens to let food pass into the stomach and shuts to stop acid and other stomach contents from returning to the esophagus. One typical component of GERD is LES dysfunction, which causes stomach acid to reflux into the esophagus and cause pain and irritation.

The Role Of The Esophagus And Lower Esophageal Sphincter (Les)

Food is transported from the mouth to the stomach via the esophagus, which is an important part of the digestive process. Food is propelled downhill by the synchronized contraction and relaxation of this muscular tube, a process known as peristalsis.

Since the esophagus does not have the same mucosal coating as the stomach, stomach acid might harm it.

As a valve, the Lower Esophageal Sphincter (LES) controls how much food passes down the esophagus and prevents stomach contents from flowing backward. Stomach acid stays in its proper place because, in a healthy swallowing pattern, the lower end of the LES stays closed. However, acid reflux occurs when the LES weakens or relaxes improperly, as observed in GERD, resulting in symptoms including regurgitation and heartburn.

LES dysfunction may be brought on by several things, including drugs, smoking, certain meals and drinks, and obesity. To properly manage GERD and avoid symptom flare-ups, it is essential to comprehend these triggers. In addition to drugs that strengthen the LES or lower the production of stomach acid, lifestyle adjustments including weight reduction and dietary adjustments are often advised to relieve symptoms and prevent additional harm to the esophagus.

Mechanisms Of Reflux

Acid from the stomach may flow backward into the esophagus during reflux, irritating and inflaming the lining of the esophagus. Several variables, such as LES dysfunction, elevated intra-abdominal pressure, and compromised esophageal clearance, contribute to this process.

When a person has GERD, their LES may weaken or relax improperly, letting stomach acid leak into their esophagus. Caffeine, alcohol, and fatty or spicy meals may all worsen LES relaxation, which increases the likelihood that reflux will develop. Pregnancy and obesity may also raise intra-abdominal pressure, which pushes stomach contents upward and exacerbates reflux symptoms.

Patients with GERD have worsening reflux due to impaired esophageal clearance, which is the esophagus's inability to remove material refluxed back into the stomach. The acid may remain in the esophagus and worsen symptoms due to conditions such as delayed gastric emptying, hiatal hernia, and esophageal dysmotility.

Comprehending the processes causing reflux is essential to customizing treatment plans that target the root causes of gastroesophageal reflux disease. Medication to enhance esophageal clearance and lower acid production, together with lifestyle changes targeted at decreasing LES relaxation and intra-abdominal pressure, are essential for controlling reflux symptoms and averting GERD-related problems.

CHAPTER 3

Lifestyle Modifications For Managing Gerd

Dietary Changes: Foods To Avoid And Foods To Include

An important factor in controlling GERD symptoms is diet. While certain meals might assist reduce pain, others can either cause or exacerbate acid reflux. Knowing what to put in and remove from your diet may make a big difference in your quality of life.

Foods to Steer Clear of:

1. Spicy Foods: Foods that are spicy may irritate the esophagus and increase the production of acid, which can cause pain and heartburn. It is advisable to restrict or stay away from meals that include chili powder, hot peppers, and other spicy substances.

2. Acidic Foods: Acidic foods include tomatoes, citrus fruits and juices, and dressings made with vinegar, which may worsen GERD symptoms. The lower esophageal sphincter may be weakened by certain meals, reopening the door for stomach acid to reflux into the esophagus.

3. Fatty Foods: Eating a lot of fat may slow down digestion and increase acid production in the stomach. Eat in moderation or stay away from fried meals, fatty meats, and creamy sauces.

4. Carbonated Drinks: Soda and other carbonated beverages may raise stomach pressure and cause acid reflux. Drink less carbonated beverages and more water or herbal tea to lower your chance of heartburn.

5. Chocolate and Mint: The compound methylxanthines found in chocolate can relax the lower esophageal sphincter, resulting in reflux.

Additionally, mint may loosen the sphincter and exacerbate symptoms in some people.

Foods to Add:

1. Lean Proteins: Include foods like beans, fish, and chicken in your diet as lean sources of protein. When compared to fatty meat cuts, these alternatives are less likely to cause acid reflux.

2. Complex Carbohydrates: For those with GERD, whole grains like oatmeal, brown rice, and whole wheat bread are great options. They provide nutrition and fiber without aggravating reflux symptoms.

3. Non-acidic Fruits: Low-acid fruits like bananas, apples, and melons are usually well-tolerated, while citrus fruits should be avoided. These fruits don't irritate the esophagus offering vital vitamins and minerals.

4. Veggies: A lot of veggies are low in acidity and fat, which makes them a good choice for meals that are GERD-friendly. Include a range of vibrant veggies in your diet to guarantee proper nourishment.

5. Low-fat Dairy: Choose dairy products like yogurt and skim milk that are low-fat or fat-free. These choices provide you with protein and calcium without aggravating your acid reflux symptoms.

Importance Of Weight Management

Keeping a healthy weight is essential for controlling the symptoms of GERD. Overweight may exacerbate reflux by putting more pressure on the stomach, particularly in the belly. People with GERD may lessen the intensity and frequency of their symptoms by decreasing weight via diet and exercise.

How Losing Weight Benefits:

1. Lessens Pressure on the Stomach: Obesity may put pressure on the stomach, causing acid reflux into the esophagus. Reduction of body weight may relieve this pressure and lessen the chance of reflux.

2. Enhances Esophageal Function: Reduced lower esophageal sphincter tone and reduced motility are two alterations in esophageal function that are linked to obesity. Losing weight may lessen GERD symptoms and help restore normal esophageal function.

3. Reduces Inflammation: Chronic inflammation, which may aggravate GERD symptoms and cause esophageal damage, is associated with obesity. All across the body, including the esophagus, inflammation may be decreased by losing weight.

4. Enhances Response to Treatment: Losing weight may make GERD drugs and other therapies more effective. A healthy weight may result in a reduction in medicine dosages or more symptom alleviation for the affected person.

Tips For Eating And Drinking

Simple dietary and drinking adjustments may have a big impact on how well your GERD symptoms are managed. You may reduce reflux episodes and enhance your general quality of life by implementing these suggestions.

Tips for Eating:

1. Eat More Often and in Smaller Portions: Eating large meals might cause the stomach to expand and raise the chance of reflux. Instead, to avoid too much stomach distention, choose smaller servings spaced out throughout the day.

2. Refrain from Eating Right Before Bed: Give yourself at least two to three hours to recover from your meal before dozing off. Because of this, there is a decreased chance of reflux throughout the night and gravity may assist keep stomach acid in the stomach.

3. Chew Carefully: Give food a good chewing experience before swallowing. This lessens the chance of reflux by promoting digestion and lessening the strain on the stomach.

4. Eat Sitting Upright: To avoid putting strain on the stomach, sit upright and maintain proper posture. Rather than slouching on the couch or in bed, sit up straight at a table.

Tips for Drinking:

1. Water is the greatest beverage option for those who have GERD, so stay hydrated.

To keep hydrated throughout the day without aggravating reflux symptoms, sip plenty of water.

2. Limit Your Alcohol Consumption: Drinking too much alcohol may cause reflux by relaxing the lower esophageal sphincter and producing more stomach acid. Avoid or use alcohol in moderation, particularly just before bed.

3. Select Non-acidic drinks: Decaffeinated coffee, herbal tea, and non-citrus fruit juices are examples of non-acidic drinks. These drinks are less likely to cause reflux than fizzy or acidic beverages.

4. Use a Straw: To reduce contact between the teeth and esophagus while consuming acidic liquids such as orange or tomato juice, use a straw. This may lessen the chance of inflammation and erosion.

Through the adoption of these lifestyle changes, people with GERD may better control their symptoms and enhance their general health.

CHAPTER 4

Medications For Gerd

Over-The-Counter Antacids

OTC antacids are comparable to the front-line combatants in the fight against GERD pain. By neutralizing stomach acid, they quickly relieve symptoms such as indigestion, heartburn, and sour stomach. These drugs usually include chemicals like aluminum hydroxide, magnesium hydroxide, or calcium carbonate that react with the excess acid in your stomach to produce water and other neutral substances.

Antacids' quick action is one of their main benefits. Within minutes of consumption, they may begin to relieve the burning feeling that is often linked to acid reflux. Nevertheless, compared to other GERD drugs, their effects are rather fleeting, often lasting between thirty and sixty minutes. Because of this, rather than being a long-term treatment for persistent GERD, they are often used as a band-aid for minor or sporadic symptoms.

It's crucial to remember that antacids only treat the symptoms of GERD; they don't treat the underlying cause or stop it from coming back. For more thorough treatment of the condition, they work best when combined with other medications or lifestyle changes. Antacids can also interact with some prescription drugs or cause negative side effects in people with certain medical conditions, so it's important to see a doctor before taking them regularly.

H2 Receptor Blockers

Another class of drugs that are frequently used to treat GERD is called H2 receptor blockers, or H2 antagonists.

This class of drugs is especially useful when the disease's symptoms are more severe or persistent. These medications function by preventing histamine from acting on the stomach's histamine H2 receptors, which lowers the production of stomach acid.

H2 receptor blockers that are commonly used include cimetidine (Tagamet), nizatidine (Axid), ranitidine (Zantac), and famotidine (Pepcid). Both over-the-counter and prescription versions are available, with higher dosages usually recommended for more severe GERD cases.

H2 receptor blockers can aid in the healing of the esophageal lining that has been harmed by acid reflux in addition to effectively treating symptoms like regurgitation and heartburn. As opposed to antacids, which relieve symptoms quickly but only temporarily, H2 blockers provide longer-lasting symptom relief, with effects that persist for several hours following each dosage.

H2 receptor blockers are generally safe for most people, but some people may experience side effects like headache, dizziness, diarrhea, and constipation. Long-term use of these drugs may also be linked to uncommon but severe side effects, like an increased risk of certain infections or a vitamin B12 deficiency. As a result, it's critical to use them under a doctor's supervision and to keep an eye out for any possible complications.

Proton Pump Inhibitors (Ppis)

When it comes to treating GERD, proton pump inhibitors (PPIs) are thought to be the best option, particularly for those who have more severe or frequent symptoms or have not responded well to other treatments. These medications function by permanently inhibiting the parietal cells of the stomach's proton pump (H+/K+ ATPase), which dramatically lowers the amount of gastric acid produced.

PPIs come in prescription and over-the-counter forms. A few examples of OTC PPIs are rabeprazole (Aciphex), pantoprazole (Protonix), lansoprazole (Prevacid), and omeprazole (Prilosec). Usually taken once a day before meals, the precise dosage and timing may change based on the needs of the patient and the severity of their symptoms.

PPIs' strong and long-lasting acid-suppressive properties are one of their key benefits; they can significantly reduce GERD symptoms and speed the healing of esophageal damage brought on by repeated acid exposure. PPIs, when compared to other medications, are often found to provide better symptom control, which enables patients to live longer and experience fewer disruptions from acid reflux.

Like any medication, PPIs have some possible side effects, though. Extended usage of these medications has been linked to several adverse effects, such as a higher chance of bone breaks, deficiency in certain vitamins and minerals (like calcium, magnesium, and vitamin B12), and a higher risk of infections, especially in those with compromised immune systems. As a result, it's critical to use PPIs carefully, under a doctor's supervision, and to assess the risks and benefits of each specific situation.

In conclusion, drugs are an essential part of the treatment of GERD because they reduce symptoms and encourage the repair of esophageal damage. Proton pump inhibitors are very good at long-term acid production suppression, H2 receptor blockers offer more sustained symptom control, and over-the-counter antacids provide fast but temporary relief.

People with GERD can successfully manage their illness and enhance their quality of life by being aware of how each type of medication functions and collaborating closely with a healthcare professional to determine the best course of action.

CHAPTER 5

Surgical Options For Gerd

Fundoplication Surgery

One surgical technique that is frequently used to treat gastroesophageal reflux disease (GERD) is fundoplication surgery. To strengthen the lower esophageal sphincter (LES) and stop stomach acid from flowing back into the esophagus, the fundus, or upper portion of the stomach, is wrapped around the lower part of the esophagus.

A laparoscope, a thin tube with a camera attached, is used by the surgeon to guide small incisions made in the abdomen during fundoplication surgery. Compared to open surgery, this minimally invasive method shortens recovery times and eases pain after surgery.

The fundus of the stomach is carefully wrapped around the esophagus by the surgeon, forming a structure that functions as a valve to stop acid reflux. Heartburn, regurgitation, and chest pain are among the symptoms of GERD that this procedure effectively relieves.

Following fundoplication surgery, patients might feel uncomfortable for a few days and have trouble swallowing. But most people can resume their regular activities in a week or two. To promote appropriate healing and reduce complications, it is crucial to adhere to the post-operative instructions given by the medical staff.

Although fundoplication surgery is usually safe, there are risks associated with it, just like with any surgical procedure, including bleeding, infection, and anesthesia-related complications. Before making a choice, patients should speak with their healthcare provider about the advantages and disadvantages of the surgery.

Endoscopic Treatments

For the management of GERD, endoscopic procedures provide less invasive options than traditional surgery. An endoscope, a flexible tube that is inserted through the mouth and into the esophagus and has a camera and other instruments attached, is used to perform these procedures.

Stretta therapy is a popular endoscopic treatment for gastric reflux disease. The lower esophageal sphincter and the esophageal muscles receive radiofrequency energy during Stretta therapy, which causes them to thicken and strengthen. This lessens acid reflux and enhances LES functionality.

The insertion of a LINX device is an additional endoscopic treatment choice. A small, flexible ring made of magnetic beads is called the LINX device, and it is wrapped around the lower esophagus. Food and liquids can pass through the LES normally while acid reflux is prevented thanks to the beads' magnetic attraction.

The majority of endoscopic GERD treatments are well tolerated, and they can be done as outpatient procedures, allowing patients to return home the same day of the procedure. Most people recover quickly and can return to their regular activities in a matter of days.

Even though endoscopic procedures have several benefits over surgery, not everyone with GERD may benefit from them. Choosing the right patient is essential to choosing the best course of treatment. To decide on the best course of action, patients must have a complete evaluation and talk through their options with a surgeon or gastroenterologist.

Patient Selection And Risks

Choosing the right patient is essential to figuring out the best course of treatment for GERD. It is important to consider factors like the severity of symptoms, underlying medical conditions, and patient preferences when treating patients with GERD, as not all of them are candidates for surgery or endoscopic treatments.

Typically, patients who are candidates for fundoplication surgery have moderate to severe GERD symptoms that are not sufficiently managed by medication or lifestyle changes. Additionally, they might have GERD-related complications like Barrett's esophagus or esophageal strictures, which call for surgery.

Patients who prefer less invasive options or who have milder GERD symptoms may benefit more from endoscopic treatments. However, not every patient is a good candidate for endoscopic procedures; it's important to take into account things like the esophageal size and shape, the existence of a hiatal hernia, and prior surgical experience.

The risks and complications associated with surgical and endoscopic treatments for GERD are similar to those associated with any medical procedure. Infection, bleeding, stomach or esophageal perforations, and unfavorable reactions to anesthesia or drugs are a few examples of these.

Patients must consult with their healthcare provider about the possible risks and benefits of various treatment options to make an informed decision that takes into account their unique needs and preferences. The best course of treatment for each patient can be decided with the assistance of a surgeon or gastroenterologist who will perform a thorough evaluation.

CHAPTER 6

Complications Of Untreated Gerd

Esophagitis And Barrett's Esophagus

The term "esophagitis" refers to inflammation of the lining of the esophagus and is a common consequence of untreated GERD. Constant exposure to stomach acid causes inflammation of the esophageal tissue, which can result in erosions or ulcers, as well as redness and swelling. Severe cases of this condition may result in bleeding, discomfort, pain, and difficulty swallowing.

If GERD is not treated, a more serious complication called Barrett's esophagus may eventually develop. It happens when aberrant cells that resemble those in the intestine replace the healthy cells lining the lower esophagus. Prolonged exposure to acid reflux causes a change known as metaplasia.

Although most people with Barrett's esophagus do not develop cancer, having the condition increases the risk of developing esophageal cancer.

Esophagitis and Barrett's esophagus require close observation and ongoing care. Both lifestyle modifications like cutting back on trigger foods, sleeping with the head of the bed raised, and taking medication to lower acid production can help relieve symptoms and stop more esophageal damage. Sometimes, to treat problems or lower the risk of cancer, treatments like endoscopy or surgery are advised.

Strictures And Ulcers

Rigidity and ulcers in the esophagus can also result from untreated GERD. The narrowing of the esophagus caused by scar tissue formation as a result of acid reflux injury and chronic inflammation is known as a stricture.

Treating this narrowing may be necessary to widen the esophagus and alleviate symptoms, as it can make swallowing challenging.

Open sores called ulcers arise in the lining of the esophagus due to prolonged irritation and inflammation caused by stomach acid. These ulcers may hurt, bleed, or make swallowing difficult. They may result in complications like bleeding or esophageal perforation if untreated.

Combining medication to lessen acid production and encourage healing with lifestyle changes to stop further damage is a common treatment for strictures and ulcers. In extreme situations, treatments like surgery or esophageal dilatation (widening) might be required to treat strictures or heal ulcers.

Respiratory Complications

Several respiratory problems, such as asthma, a persistent cough, and recurrent pneumonia, can result from GERD. Stomach acid can cause irritation and inflammation when it refluxes into the esophagus and enters the lungs and airways.

When GERD patients have acid reflux, their airway inflammation and bronchospasm can worsen their asthma symptoms. Another common respiratory GERD complication is chronic cough, which is caused by stomach acid reflux irritating the throat and inducing cough reflexes.

Since GERD symptoms can sometimes mimic those of other respiratory disorders, diagnosing GERD-related respiratory complications can be difficult in certain situations. GERD treatment, however, can frequently alleviate respiratory symptoms and lessen the frequency and intensity of respiratory infections, coughing fits, and asthma attacks.

A combination of drugs to lessen acid reflux, inhalers or other medications to control asthma symptoms, and lifestyle changes to minimize reflux episodes may be used to manage the respiratory complications of GERD. When other treatments are ineffective for severe reflux or other complications, surgery may be advised in certain circumstances.

In general, it is essential to diagnose and treat GERD as soon as possible to avoid complications and enhance quality of life. People with GERD can lower their risk of developing complications like respiratory issues, strictures, ulcers, esophagitis, Barrett's esophagus, and strictures by managing their condition regularly and working with healthcare professionals.

CHAPTER 7

Gerd In Special Populations

Gerd In Pregnancy

The body changes significantly during pregnancy to make room for the developing fetus, and these changes can occasionally cause the onset or aggravation of gastroesophageal reflux disease (GERD). Hormonal changes, especially the rise in progesterone levels, are a major cause of GERD during pregnancy. The lower esophageal sphincter (LES), which typically serves as a barrier between the stomach and the esophagus, is one of the muscles that progesterone relaxes. Because of this, the LES may become weaker and permit stomach acid to reflux up into the esophagus, leading to heartburn and other GERD symptoms.

Moreover, the uterus's growth during pregnancy may put pressure on the stomach, which exacerbates acid reflux. Additionally, this pressure may force stomach contents upward, aggravating symptoms. Furthermore, eating habits that exacerbate reflux, like eating larger meals or consuming specific foods, can exacerbate symptoms of gastroparesis.

A mix of lifestyle changes and, occasionally, medication is used to treat GERD during pregnancy. It's common knowledge that pregnant women should eat smaller, more frequent meals to ease the strain on their stomachs and steer clear of acidic or spicy foods. To prevent reflux during the night, it's also advised to avoid lying down right after eating and to raise the head of the bed while you sleep.

Pregnancy-related GERD medication is usually restricted because of worries about possible harm to the growing fetus.

Heartburn can be momentarily relieved by taking antacids that contain calcium or magnesium, and they are frequently regarded as safe. To ensure the safety of the mother and the unborn child, a healthcare professional must be consulted before commencing any medication regimen during pregnancy.

Gerd In Children

Pediatric patients with gastroesophageal reflux disease (GERD) range in age from newborns to teenagers. Gastroesophageal reflux disease (GERD) in infants is commonly referred to as infant reflux or GER. Babies frequently have this condition because of how immature their digestive systems are. Infant reflux usually goes away on its own as the baby's digestive system develops. On the other hand, some newborns may experience reflux disease (GERD), which is defined by frequent, continuous episodes of reflux that hurt or result in complications.

Infants with GERD frequently spit up, get agitated during or after feedings, arch their backs, and gain little weight. GERD symptoms in older kids and teenagers can include reflux, chest pain, difficulty swallowing, heartburn, and persistent cough.

Children with GERD are typically diagnosed using a combination of clinical assessment, medical history, and diagnostic testing. Medication, dietary adjustments, and lifestyle changes may all be part of the treatment for pediatric GERD. Feeding adjustments for infants with GERD, such as thickening breast milk or formula, feeding them upright during and after, and giving them smaller, more frequent feedings, may help lessen reflux episodes.

A vital part of managing GERD in older children and adolescents is making lifestyle changes like cutting back on trigger foods, eating smaller meals, and keeping a healthy weight. Proton pump inhibitors (PPIs) and H2-receptor antagonists are two more drugs that doctors may prescribe to treat symptoms and lower stomach acid production. Surgical intervention might be taken into consideration in extreme situations or when problems develop.

Gerd In The Elderly

The prevalence of GERD tends to rise with age, and symptoms and complications associated with GERD are more common in the elderly. Reduced LES pressure and esophageal motility are two alterations in the gastrointestinal tract that are linked to aging and may play a role in the onset or aggravation of GERD.

Moreover, GERD risk can be further increased by comorbidities that are frequently observed in the elderly population, such as obesity, hiatal hernias, and medications that relax the LES or increase stomach acid production.

Due to overlapping symptoms with other conditions common in this age group, such as heart disease or gastritis, diagnosing GERD in the elderly can be difficult. Elderly people may also report atypical symptoms like coughing, hoarseness, or throat clearing more frequently than typical symptoms like heartburn.

A multidisciplinary approach is often necessary for the management of GERD in the elderly. This approach includes addressing underlying comorbidities, making dietary and lifestyle modifications, and managing medication. Proton pump inhibitors (PPIs) and H2-receptor antagonists may be prescribed in certain situations to lessen the production of stomach acid and relieve symptoms.

In formulating a GERD treatment plan, it is imperative to take the individual requirements and medical background of senior patients into account. To guarantee the efficacy of treatment and avoid consequences linked to untreated GERD, like Barrett's esophagus or esophageal strictures, routine monitoring and follow-up are essential.

CHAPTER 8

Managing Gerd Symptoms

Tips For Nighttime Heartburn Relief

Heartburn at night can be especially bothersome to sleep and general well-being. The following are some doable methods to reduce heartburn at night and enhance sleep:

1. Raise Your Upper Extremities:

When you sleep, you can lessen the likelihood that stomach acid will reflux into your esophagus by raising the head of your bed by six to eight inches. Blocks placed beneath the bedposts or bed risers can be used to accomplish this.

2. Prevent Eating Late at Night:

Avoid having substantial meals or heavy snacks right before bed. Stomach acid is produced during food digestion, which can worsen heartburn symptoms while you're sleeping.

3. Adjust Your Position While Sleeping:

Heartburn during the night can be lessened by sleeping on your left side. This posture lowers the risk of acid reflux by keeping your stomach below your esophagus.

4. Keep an Eye on Your Prescriptions:

Several drugs, including those for depression, high blood pressure, and asthma, can exacerbate the symptoms of GERD. To discuss any alternatives or changes to your medication regimen, speak with your healthcare provider.

5. Determine Food Triggers:

Keep a record of the foods and drinks that often make you feel like you have heartburn, especially after dark.

Caffeine, alcohol, citrus fruits, and spicy food are common triggers. Preventing these triggers before going to bed can help lessen heartburn during the night.

6. Utilize relaxation techniques:

Stress can make GERD symptoms worse, including heartburn that occurs at night. Before going to bed, practice relaxation techniques like deep breathing, meditation, or gentle yoga to help you unwind and lower your stress levels.

Coping With Regurgitation And Chest Pain

Common signs of gastric reflux disease (GERD) include regurgitation, chest pain, and the feeling that acid is backing up into your mouth or throat. The following are some effective coping mechanisms for these symptoms:

1. Sustain a Healthy Weight:

Gaining too much weight can put a strain on your stomach, increasing regurgitation and reflux. Maintaining a healthy weight and lowering GERD symptoms can be achieved by following an exercise regimen and eating well.

2. Put on loose-fitting attire:

Chest pain and regurgitation are two symptoms of GERD that can be made worse by wearing tight clothing, especially around the waist and abdomen. Choose loose-fitting apparel to ease discomfort and lessen pressure on your stomach.

3. Steer clear of trigger foods:

For those who have GERD, certain foods and drinks, like chocolate, peppermint, fried or fatty foods, and carbonated drinks, can cause regurgitation and chest pain. To reduce symptoms, recognize these triggers and stay away from them.

4. Consume More Often and Smaller Meals:

Eating large meals can worsen the symptoms of GERD by putting more pressure on the stomach. Instead, to avoid overtaxing your digestive system, choose smaller, more frequent meals spread out throughout the day.

5. Maintain Proper Posture:

By applying pressure to your belly, poor posture, such as slouching or hunching over, may aggravate chest discomfort and regurgitation. To help with symptoms, sit and stand with proper posture.

6. Maintain Hydration:

Water consumption might help lower stomach acid production and lessen the intensity of GERD symptoms, such as regurgitation and chest discomfort, throughout the day. Make it a daily goal to consume eight glasses of water or more.

Alleviating Throat Symptoms

For those who have GERD, throat symptoms including clearing their throat, hoarseness, and painful throat may be upsetting. Here are some efficient methods for reducing throat symptoms:

1. Steer clear of irritants:

Steer clear of irritants including air pollution, cigarette smoke, and strong chemical smells since they might aggravate GERD-related throat discomfort.

2. Maintain Hydration:

Drinking plenty of liquids, particularly water, may aid in the healing process and relieve sore throats. For added comfort, choose warm liquids like broths or herbal teas.

3. Employ a Humidifier:

Hoarseness and sore throats may be made worse by dry air. You may relieve your sore throat by adding moisture to the air in your bedroom by using a humidifier.

4. Maintain Proper Oral Hygiene:

To lower the risk of infection and inflammation, practicing excellent oral hygiene, which includes brushing and flossing regularly, may help prevent bacterial development in the mouth and throat.

5. Avert Clearing Your Throat:

Recurrent cleaning of the throat might aggravate the lining and make symptoms worse. To ease pain, consider swallowing or drinking water rather than clearing your throat.

6. Think About Over-the-Counter Treatments:

Cough drops, throat sprays, and over-the-counter throat lozenges may all provide momentary relief from GERD-related throat discomfort. Seek for items with calming components like honey or menthol.

CHAPTER 9

Integrative Approaches To Gerd Management

Supplements and Herbal Remedies

Herbal treatments and supplements provide a natural approach to GERD management that many people find attractive. Without the possible negative effects of prescription drugs, these treatments may help reduce symptoms and support overall digestive health.

Slick elm, which is made from the inner bark of the slippery elm tree, is a well-liked herbal treatment for GERD. Mucilage, which is found in slippery elm, coats and calms the digestive system to relieve inflammation and discomfort. It may be taken as lozenges, capsules, or teas, among other forms. Marshmallow root is another herb that is often used to treat GERD. It has mucilage and may help reduce esophageal irritation.

Another plant that helps the digestive system and may lessen GERD symptoms is ginger. Due to its inherent anti-inflammatory qualities, it helps facilitate better digestion by speeding up food passage through the stomach. You may drink ginger tea, eat it raw, or take it as a supplement.

Furthermore, by supporting a balanced population of gut bacteria, supplements like probiotics might help manage GERD. Probiotics support the integrity of the intestinal lining and may lessen gastrointestinal tract inflammation, both of which may aid with GERD symptoms.

Before beginning any herbal cures or supplements, you should speak with a healthcare provider, particularly if you're using medication or have underlying medical issues.

Even while many herbal medicines are typically harmless, if used incorrectly, they might worsen some health concerns or interfere with drugs.

Stress Reduction Techniques

Stress is recognized to be a cause of gastric reflux disease (GERD) symptoms since it may raise stomach acid production and worsen intestinal inflammation. Thus, treating GERD may benefit from including stress-reduction strategies into your everyday routine.

Deep breathing exercises are one useful method for reducing stress. By triggering the body's relaxation response, deep breathing eases tension in the muscles and fosters serenity. Spend a few minutes each day engaging in deep breathing exercises, with an emphasis on slow, deep breaths to help reduce tension and anxiety.

Mindfulness meditation is another beneficial method. Being mindful entails focusing on the here and now without passing judgment, which helps lessen stress-inducing thoughts and anxieties. To help you relax and reduce stress, set aside sometime each day to practice mindfulness meditation. During this time, you may concentrate on your breath or your body's sensations.

Another great method for reducing stress that might help people with GERD is yoga. Yoga integrates breathing exercises, physical postures, and meditation to enhance general well-being and encourage relaxation. Some yoga positions, such as slow stretches and twists, may ease physical stress and aid in a healthy digestive system.

Together with these methods, frequent exercise, getting enough sleep, and taking part in fun activities may all help lower overall stress levels, which in turn can help control the symptoms of GERD.

Alternative Therapies

Several alternative treatments, in addition to herbal medicines and stress-reduction methods, may provide help for those with GERD.

To encourage healing and boost energy flow, acupuncture is a traditional Chinese medical procedure that involves inserting tiny needles into certain body locations. According to some research, acupuncture may reduce the symptoms of GERD by controlling the formation of stomach acid and enhancing esophageal function.

Another complementary treatment that may help people with GERD is chiropractic care. Chiropractic care focuses on musculoskeletal and spine alignment to enhance general health and well-being. Spinal misalignments may impair nerve transmission and aggravate digestive disorders like GERD. Chiropractic adjustments may assist enhance nerve function and lessen GERD symptoms by realigning the spine.

Additionally, by encouraging relaxation, easing muscular tension, and enhancing circulation, massage treatment may help manage the symptoms of GERD. Abdominal and Swedish massages are two examples of massage treatments that may help reduce stress and tension in the body, which can exacerbate symptoms of GERD.

While some GERD sufferers may find relief with alternative remedies, it's important to speak with a healthcare provider before beginning any new treatment regimen, particularly if you're on medication or have underlying medical issues.

CHAPTER 10:

Preventing Gerd Flare-Ups And Long-Term Management

Developing A Personalized Management Plan

Developing a customized GERD treatment plan requires knowing the specific triggers, symptoms, and lifestyle choices that lead to flare-ups. Together, you and your healthcare practitioner will create a strategy that is specific to your requirements.

First of all, it's important to identify triggers. These may differ from person to person, but they often consist of certain meals, drinks, pastimes, and drugs. Maintaining a food journal might assist you in identifying certain triggers so you can either stay away from them or eat them sparingly.

Medication administration is another important factor. Proton pump inhibitors (PPIs), H2 receptor blockers, and antacids are among the drugs your doctor may recommend to lower acid production or neutralize stomach acid. It's important to take these drugs as directed and to let your doctor know right away if you have any adverse effects or concerns.

For GERD management, lifestyle changes are essential in addition to medicine. This entails keeping a healthy weight, staying away from constricting apparel that puts extra strain on the belly, raising the head of your bed to lessen reflux at night, and refraining from laying down for at least three hours after eating.

Furthermore, GERD symptoms may be greatly impacted by dietary modifications. Caffeine, chocolate, citrus fruits, spicy cuisine, and fatty or fried meals are examples of common trigger foods. You may lessen the likelihood of flare-ups by limiting or eliminating certain trigger foods and switching to a diet high in fruits, vegetables, lean meats, and healthy grains.

Moreover, maintaining healthy eating habits might aid in the management of GERD. This entails digesting food completely, eating smaller, more frequent meals, and refraining from eating too rapidly. Furthermore, it's critical to maintain proper hydration throughout the day by consuming plenty of water.

Last but not least, practicing stress-reduction methods like yoga, meditation, and deep breathing exercises might help lower stress levels, which can worsen GERD symptoms. Including these methods in your daily routine may help with symptom management and general well-being.

You may successfully control GERD and enhance your quality of life by creating a specific management plan that takes into account triggers, medication, lifestyle changes, dietary adjustments, eating habits, and stress management.

Follow-Up Care And Monitoring

To guarantee the effectiveness of therapy and avoid complications, controlling GERD requires routine follow-up care and monitoring.

Following the start of therapy, your doctor will arrange follow-up visits to evaluate your progress, change your medication if needed, and answer any questions or concerns you may have. These consultations enable continuing assessments of drug tolerance and symptom management.

Your doctor could also suggest further diagnostic tests or procedures during follow-up appointments to keep an eye on your health and assess the efficacy of your therapy. These might involve esophageal manometry, pH monitoring, or endoscopy to evaluate esophageal function and identify any problems such as Barrett's esophagus or esophagitis.

Effective treatment also requires that you keep an eye on your symptoms and record any changes or flare-ups. By keeping a symptom journal, you may see trends, triggers, and opportunities for improvement, which will allow you to modify your treatment regimen as needed.

Important components of long-term treatment include lifestyle changes and drug adherence in addition to medical follow-up. To support you in managing stress, adhering to dietary and behavioral guidelines, and leading a healthy lifestyle, your healthcare practitioner may provide you with continuing education and assistance.

Furthermore, it's important to be open and honest with your healthcare provider about any changes in your symptoms, any adverse effects from your medicine, and any worries you may have. You will get individualized treatment and assistance that is tailored to your requirements thanks to our cooperation.

To successfully manage GERD and avoid problems, it is important to combine medication adherence, lifestyle adjustments, routine follow-up treatment, and open communication with your healthcare practitioner.

Living Well With Gerd: Tips For Long-Term Health

Making lifestyle changes and embracing healthy behaviors are essential to living well with gastric reflux disease (GERD) to reduce symptoms and enhance overall quality of life.

Keeping a healthy weight is one of the most crucial parts of living well with GERD.

Being overweight puts additional strain on the belly, which makes reflux symptoms worse and more frequent. You may lower your risk of GERD flare-ups by reaching and maintaining a healthy weight with a balanced diet and consistent exercise.

Additionally, minimizing symptoms may be achieved by being mindful of your food choices. Reflux may be minimized by eating smaller, more frequent meals and avoiding big ones, particularly just before bed. To help with digestion, it's also critical to chew food well and refrain from eating too rapidly.

Furthermore, controlling the symptoms of GERD may be greatly aided by wise food decisions. Flare-ups may be avoided by avoiding trigger foods including chocolate, citrus fruits, coffee, spicy and fried meals, and fatty foods. Rather, concentrate on increasing the amount of fruits, vegetables, lean meats, and whole grains in your diet.

Additionally, addressing your sleeping patterns and posture might help reduce discomfort. Refrain from leaning over or laying down just after eating as this might exacerbate reflux. Reflux throughout the night may also be avoided by raising the head of your bed by six to eight inches.

Stress reduction methods, in addition to dietary changes, may help control GERD symptoms. Practicing relaxation methods such as deep breathing exercises, meditation, and yoga may help lower stress levels, which can increase reflux symptoms.

Lastly, it's crucial to stick to your drug regimen and attend frequent follow-up meetings with your healthcare professional. Medications such as proton pump inhibitors (PPIs) or H2 receptor blockers may be recommended to lower acid production and improve symptoms. Keeping note of your symptoms and discussing them honestly with your healthcare practitioner will help ensure that your treatment plan is successful and personalized to your requirements.

By implementing these recommendations into your daily routine and adopting healthy lifestyle choices, you may successfully control GERD and enhance your overall quality of life.

CONCLUSION

In conclusion, Gastroesophageal Reflux Disease (GERD) is a chronic disorder defined by the frequent reflux of stomach acid into the esophagus, producing numerous symptoms such as heartburn, regurgitation, chest discomfort, and trouble swallowing. Throughout our investigation of GERD, many essential aspects have emerged.

Firstly, lifestyle alterations play a key part in reducing GERD symptoms. Simple modifications such as avoiding trigger foods, keeping a healthy weight, raising the head of the bed, and stopping smoking may considerably ease pain and minimize the frequency of reflux episodes.

Secondly, pharmaceutical treatment is commonly applied to manage symptoms and cure esophageal damage caused by GERD. Proton pump inhibitors (PPIs), H2 receptor antagonists, and antacids are often used to lower stomach acid production and offer comfort. However, long-term use of these drugs may contain dangers and should be monitored by healthcare specialists.

Furthermore, for those with severe or chronic GERD symptoms, surgical procedures such as fundoplication or LINX device implantation may be explored to tighten the lower esophageal sphincter and prevent reflux.

Importantly, GERD may progress to problems such as Barrett's esophagus, esophageal strictures, and even esophageal cancer if left untreated. Therefore, quick diagnosis and adequate care are critical to avoid long-term problems and enhance quality of life.

In conclusion, although GERD is a common and frequently treatable ailment, it needs constant attention and care. By implementing lifestyle modifications, sticking to medication regimens, and seeking medical help when required, persons with GERD may successfully manage their symptoms and decrease the risk of consequences, enabling them to lead productive lives free from the pain of reflux.

THE END

www.ingramcontent.com/pod-product-compliance
Lightning Source LLC
Chambersburg PA
CBHW070313230526
45470CB00002B/853